"An interesting look at cracking into the field of personal training, and gaining notoriety as a fitness professional by discovering skills and characteristics not typically taught in textbooks."

Secret Skills of Personal Training

By John Izzo, BSc, NASM-CPT, PES

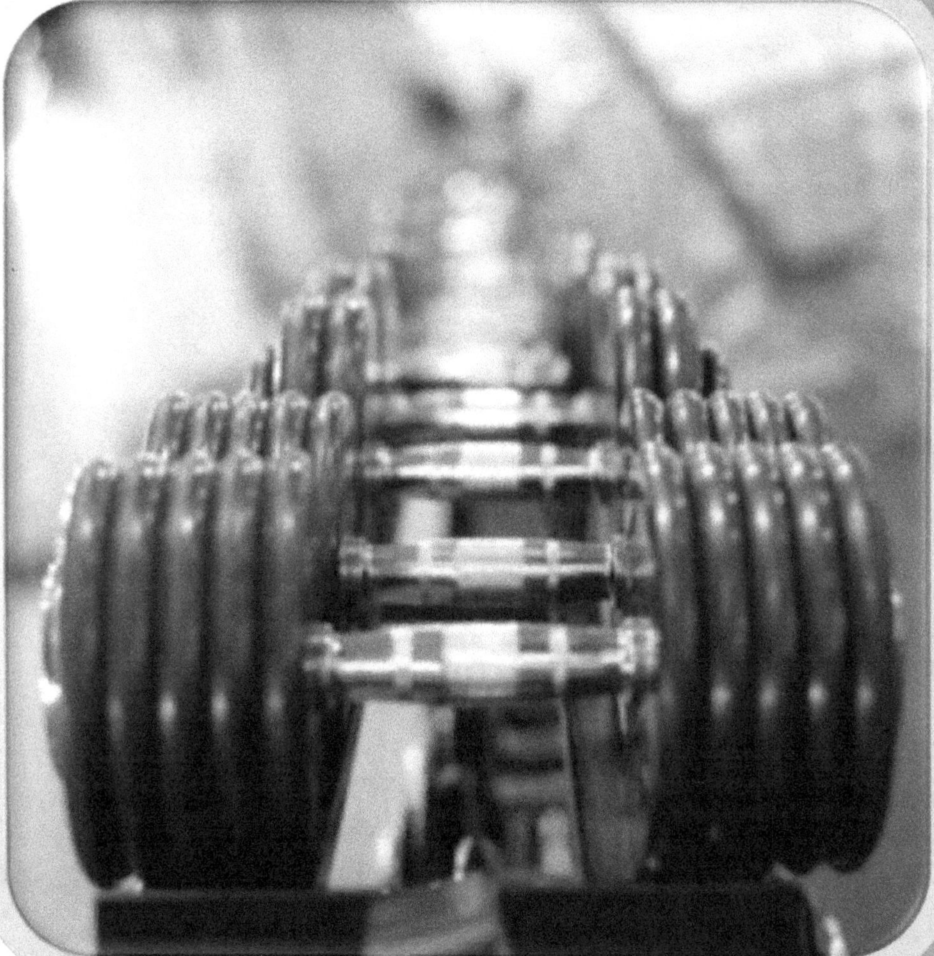

Certified Personal Trainer & Performance Enhancement Specialist

Secret Skills of Personal Training – Written by John Izzo

Disclaimer

This e-Book is copyrighted © standAPARTfitness.com and John Izzo. This e-Book may not be reproduced or transmitted by any means: electronic, mechanical, photocopying, or recorded without prior written consent by the author. The information contained in standAPARTfitness.com or its products should not be used to diagnose, treat, or cure any illness, disease, metabolic disorder, or health ailment. Participants, contributors, members, readers, visitors of standAPARTfitness.com should consult a licensed medical physician or health care provided for any aforementioned conditions. Use of the programs, products, advice, and information contained in this website or its affiliated products, links, associates is at the sole choice and risk of the reader and visitor.

Legal Notice

The material contained in this website, its products, programs, articles, text, messages, newsletters, postings, and photos is provided for educational and informational purposes only and is not intended to be or replace medical advice. Neither standAPARTfitness.com, nor its authors, administrators, affiliates, members, or associates assume any liability for the information contained herein. The information contained in standAPARTfitness.com or its products should not be used to diagnose, treat, or cure any illness, disease, metabolic disorder, or health ailment. Participants, contributors, members, readers, visitors of standAPARTfitness.com should consult a licensed medical physician or health care provided for any aforementioned conditions. Use of the programs, products, advice, and information contained in this website or its affiliated products, links, associates is at the sole choice and risk of the reader and visitor.

Copyright

Without limiting the rights under the copyright reserved above, no part of this publication and/or website (including the title standAPARTfitness.com or its logo) may be reproduced, stored, or introduced into a retrieval system, or transmitted, in any form or by any means (electronic, mechanical, photocopying, recording, or otherwise), without the prior written consent of the author. Use of the websites name, title, logo, products, or publications without prior written consent is illegal and punishable by law.

Terms of Service

THE INFORMATION CONTAINED HEREIN IS PROVIDED "AS-IS", "AS AVAILABLE" AND ALL WARRANTIES, EXPRESSED OR IMPLIED, ARE DISCLAIMED (INCLUDING BUT NOT LIMITED TO THE DISCLAIMER OF ANY IMPLIED WARRANTIES OF MERCHANTABILITY AND FITNESS FOR A PARTICULAR PURPOSE). THE INFORMATION AND SERVICES MAY CONTAIN BUGS, ERRORS, PROBLEMS, OR OTHER LIMITATIONS. WE AND OUR AFFILIATED PARTIES HAVE NO LIABILITY WHATSOEVER FOR YOUR USE OF ANY INFORMATION OR SERVICE. IN PARTICULAR, BUT NOT AS A LIMITATION THEREOF, WE AND OUR AFFILIATED PARTIES ARE LIABLE FOR ANY INDIRECT, SPECIAL, INCIDENTAL, OR CONSEQUENTIAL DAMAGES (INCLUDING DAMAGES FOR LOSS OF BUSINESS, LOSS OF PROFITS, LITIGATION, OR THE LIKE), WHETHER BASED ON BREACH OF CONTRACT, BREACH OF WARRANTY, TORT (INCLUDING NEGLIGENCE), PRODUCT LIABILITY OR OTHERWISE, EVEN IF ADVISED OF THE POSSIBILITY OF SUCH DAMAGES. THE NEGATION OF DAMAGES SET FORTH ABOVE ARE FUNDAMENTAL ELEMENTS OF THE BASIS OF THE BARGAIN BETWEEN YOU AND US. THIS SITE AND THE INFORMATION WOULD NOT BE PROVIDED WITHOUT SUCH LIMITATIONS. NO ADVICE OR INFORMATION, WHETHER ORAL OR WRITTEN, OBTAINED BY YOU FROM US THROUGH THIS SITE OR E-MAIL, SHALL CREATE ANY WARRANTY, REPRESENTATION OR GUARANTEE NOT EXPRESSLY STATED IN THIS AGREEMENT.

This book is dedicated to every client I have ever encountered that had allowed me to coach them.

To all current and future clients… you'll be in my next book ☺

To the readers: Thank you for purchasing this book and allowing me to "coach" you as you take your first few steps in this wonderful career and fitness endeavor. It is truly a unique profession and one that will reward you daily.

Introduction

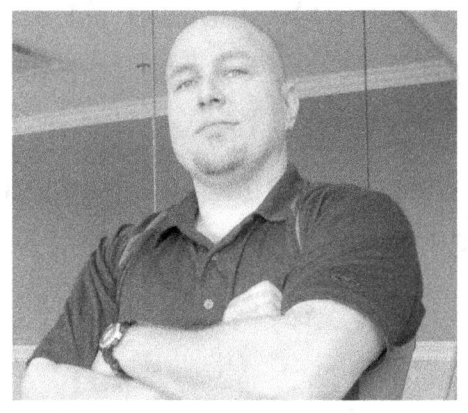

I have been asked why I wrote this book. Who am I and why should people listen to me? Well, I'll take you back a bit. My passion for fitness stems from my own personal journey to self-betterment. I have tried a million different types of exercise programs; over a hundred different supplements; and read every book I can get my hands on going as far back as 1989. I became a faithful subscriber to Joe Weider's Muscle & Fitness® and other publications since 1988. The collection of old magazines has become a pseudo-time capsule for me. My very first workout is still tacked on my attic wall dated 1990. Back then, I worked out during the hot summer months in my parent's stuffy, non-ventilated attic on equipment I built using pulley's, clothesline, and bricks purchased at the nearby tool store. My own battles with physique alteration enhanced my ability to relate to others and made me VERY comfortable in gyms. I was never as big as some of the guys in there, but I was always as strong or sometimes...stronger. Early on, I made a point to wear big, baggy shirts in commercial gyms. My goal was to fill those big, baggy shirts with MUSCLE! Something about young guys wearing tight shirts to show off the little muscles they attained. It made me feel complacent...like my goal had been reached. It's funny, but it worked. I must have run into a dozen old gym friends in the last 3 years and they have all become fat, out-of-shape husbands, or couch quarterbacks. At 35, I feel stronger and healthier than I ever have.

So, when you have these MAGNIFICENT feelings and passion about what you can accomplishment, what do you do? You share them with others! I became a successful personal trainer at EVERY club I worked for and it wasn't my physique or my bench numbers...it was my knack for busting through the mental barriers that people create and making them believe that they have the same abilities that all able-bodied humans possess. It was my ability to INSPIRE, INFLUENCE, and INSTRUCT that helped make fat people look at themselves in the mirror with hope and fire. It was my knack for relating to the high-school athlete and challenging them to a race... or taking a yoga class with a client just so she will feel comfortable. It was PASSION.

I'm not the only one that has it. You have it too because you have acquired this book and are interested in taking your passion and skills to a higher level. We all have a passion in something or many things. When you find an outlet that lets you express your passion (that outlet can be another person, house, or career) you do what you can to preserve it.

Of All the Things You Can Be

Throughout this book, I am going to challenge your position on making the choice to become a fitness professional. My intent is not to "talk you out of it", but to really make you understand what it will take to become successful and experience your passion at work on a daily basis with hundreds of people. I could sugar-coat some of my thoughts, but then that wouldn't be fair to you, as you would miss out on the directive-ness of this book's objective. So read on and simply contemplate the circumstances and tasks that I lay out.

So you want to be a personal trainer, huh? Good...let me ask why?

"Do you want to get up at 5am and drive to the gym in 15 degree temperature to train 270 pound Mrs. Fields?"

"Do you want to stay at the gym till 9pm for Rafael to meet you only to find out he cancelled his appointment at 8:30pm?"

"Do you want to train yourself after you've spent 8 hours in the gym with 8 different clients, only to have an audience watch you're every rep?"

If you answered "No" to any of the questions, than stop reading this book, stop contemplating obtaining a certification, stop buying all the new sports apparel, stop reading all your fitness magazines, and stop working out!

You are probably saying: "Huh? Stop working out?"

That's right. Stop exercising and 'getting off' on people walking up to you every day and asking for your advice and feeling like "**somebody**"!

Everyone watches your every move, every rep, every set, and everyone knows your name.

But it feels good—doesn't it? It feels good having people walk up to you in the gym and ask you:

> *"How do I use this machine?"*
>
> *"What was that exercise you were just doing?"*
>
> *"How do I get rid of this?"*

It feels good to be able to provide an answer and be recognized for all the hard work you put into your own personal fitness program. It feels exhilarating to <u>lead</u>. It's exciting to be an ambassador of something that is supposed to be good for you! Yes, it does.

Being a Leader

It feels ecstatic to be recognized as a leader...in the weight-room, in the aerobics studio, in the locker room, on the field, in the classroom, and at work. That's why we love to be personal trainers and why we strive to learn every aspect of fitness -- to be able to serve others effectively and completely. We want to help others. We want to share knowledge, experience, and support. We want to have our hard work recognized and our accomplishments duly noted. We want that shirt that says "Staff" or "Trainer" on the back and walk around the club. We want to get down on our hands and knees and spray that treadmill and wipe off all the dry sweat beads from the elliptical. We want to change those towels...carry that clipboard, re-rack those weights, and find the other handle to the cable column**....HUH?**

You're probably now saying: "I thought you were talking about helping people and being a leader?"

I AM talking about being a leader, educator, coach, instructor, and motivator. But just as comics start from scratch before they land the big venues, so do personal trainers. And this book will examine what *"to-do"* and what *"not to-do"* to break into the personal training business and **stay in it.**

History Check

I started out, much like I will detail in this book--from the bottom to the top in about 10 years. The only difference between me and you reading this right now is my love for fitness began close to 17 years ago. I grew up in dungeon weight-rooms, Boy's Clubs and YMCAs, and later "graduated" to gyms. My background is likely to be similar to the origin of your passion, so you will be able to relate to my stories. Do you need to be a "fitness junkie" to achieve status of "personal trainer"? No, but you need to learn anatomy & physiology, biomechanics, nutrition, communication, and a bunch of other stuff.

I have seen the personal training field evolve since 1993, but it has really become a serious career around 2000. Here's a little history: Back in the mid-80's-90's, personal trainers were specifically hired by the wealthy and professional athletes. In Hollywood, actors had personal trainers that usually dubbed as their stunt doubles. In bodybuilding, competitors had trainers that dubbed as their workout partners or spotters, and professional athletes looked to their strength coaches or athletic trainers (ATC) for exercise advice.

Since around 1998, the need for preventative medicine and health care woes prompted Americans to become more proactive in regards to their personal health. After waking medical health professionals from their slumber, doctors started recognizing exercise as a viable option for you to stay out of their office. And today, shows like "Biggest Loser®", "Fit-TV®", and "Survivor®" detail how important it is to become healthy, look healthy, and stay healthy.

So enough of the history lesson, how do you crack into the personal training business and gain notoriety as a fitness professional? Well let's get started.

Getting Your Feet Wet

Let's get your feet wet in the fitness field. If you are already a member of a fitness center, gym, or other club, GREAT! If not, and you are really sure you want to get into this business than you need to gain some **observational experience.** I advise purchasing a membership to an athletic facility or gym to begin step number one. Observational experience allows you to become a *"people watcher"*. That is the first and foremost important aspect to achieve a sensory skill of reading people. You need to observe people in action. If you are not a member of a club, go to your local mall or shopping plaza. Sit down on a park bench or be seated in your favorite restaurant. Take a few minutes and look around. Spend a good 10-15 minutes observing the following:

1.)Who is around you?

2.)What structures surround you?

3.)What is the ambiance in the setting? (energy levels, etc)

4.)How is the lighting?

5.) What actions are people engaged in? (sitting, talking, walking, eating, lifting, etc)

6.) What is the stature or demeanor of people around you? (Laughing, straining, anger, frustration, happiness, intuitiveness, slouching, etc.)

7.) What position are you in should you have to react if the situation dramatically changes? (fire, emergency, choking, etc)

8.) Account for the position your partner is in. (Remember, in your company, <u>a second or third person become an extension of you.</u>) (**Teaching Anchor #1**)

9.) What do you hear? Listen closely to sounds around you.

10.) Keep your eyes moving. Don't stare...observe the environment collectively. (Make glances everywhere and piece them together in your head.)

Okay, I know what you are thinking: "What does this have to do with being a personal trainer?" My answer: "LOTS". If you are going to be recognized as the "**Information Booth of Fitness**", then you need to know every aspect of what you are talking about and anticipate concerns.

"If you presently workout in a gym, between sets of each exercise, take a look around and observe people that are using the machines, cardio equipment, free weights, or are just plain 'ol socializing. Notably, if they are talking constantly they must not take their fitness goals seriously. Right?

We can assume they workout to say: "I workout".

Watch the ones that grimace and groan.

There is a reason they are straining and using a lot of weight. They desire to change. Maybe they want to be the biggest or strongest guy in the gym, at work, or home?

Watch the girl on the elliptical in her tight workout gear. She wants to be noticed for a reason. Watch the heavy-set girl who looks out of place...and probably feels it."

Once you are adequate in "observational skills", now it's time to get you involved in all these situations. Let's look for employment. I know what you are thinking:

"I don't have any experience training others."

"I'm not certified."

"I don't have a degree."

"I don't look fit."

That doesn't matter just yet. You have to be in a <u>position where you can "service others"</u> in order to fully appreciate this craft. **(This is Teaching Anchor #2)**

How do you do you that? Read on.

The Art of Dabbling

No one wakes up one day and becomes a great personal trainer. They gain experience.

Unfortunately, experience can be equated to being thrown into a *pack of wolves* or a *pack of kittens.* I am going to suggest you throw yourself in a pack of kittens for now. The wolves will come in later pages.

Obtain a job in some sort of fitness position. There are plenty of organizations that are involved with health and fitness without needing extensive qualifications. Actually, many of these facilities provide in-house training that will enable you to grow within the company and provide much-needed education to help you further your career *outside of the company.* That's right. Don't plan on staying with that first employment forever. You won't get anywhere. Initially, you are not looking to work as a personal trainer yet... You are asking to work in a gym as...*anything.*

> *"You need to be around people exercising. You need to be around the hum of treadmills, fogging mirrors, cardio sign-ups, lost and found clothes, and plates left on the floor. You need to gain "observational experience" and get paid for it!"*

There are a number of agencies or companies that will hire you at entry level into fitness service. Here are some:

YMCA's – YMCA's are notorious for hiring people off the street and educating them. YMCA's tend to look for people that follow certain personality traits that lean towards "servicing others". The YMCA provides extensive training in all fields of work—

especially health and fitness. You will most likely work as a fitness technician where you will clean equipment, conduct orientations, and interact with members. Again, this gets you around equipment and around people using the equipment.

Jewish Community Centers (JCC) – Same premise as YMCA's and other non-profit agencies. JCC's will hire you and pay you less money than a commercial gym but they don't look for the same qualifications. This is an easy way to get your foot in the door without the pressure of reaching monthly quota's and sales goals.

Town Parks & Rec's – Another great way to be around fitness junk and exercisers. Most towns don't look for certifications; they simply need a "body" to supervise the gym floor. No problem, because you are not going to stay there forever.

Women-Only facilities – I know what you are thinking. I know it is a just a small space with a bunch of hydraulic equipment, but that is not what makes them successful. They are successful because they provide results in a supportive, non-intimidating atmosphere, and you will be looked at as a special resource by these women. This is a great opportunity for you to observe support "in the flesh". These women have continuity among them. They are meshed together by the same commonalities: commitment to change and support.

Hotel Gym, School Gyms – No experts needed here, just people with supervisory skills, good judgment, and basic knowledge.

> *"Remember, I'm talking about being a personal trainer—a fitness professional—someone who has the expertise to design individualized exercise programs and back them up with proven results. A caring fitness professional can take individuals from their lowest points in life and turn them around to make them into outspoken representatives of your services.*
>
> *It doesn't happen overnight, and you'll need to be acclimated to the environment, emotions, and tools that are necessary to accomplish this."*

You're probably saying: *"This sounds like you want me to be a clipboard holding, pencil pushing, and sweat-cleaning floor attendant?"*

Yes, I do. **This is the pack of kittens**. The wolves will come later. Keep reading...

As club members see you and get to know you, they will come up to you and ask you numerous questions. Questions that you may or may not have the answer for, but it will force you to educate yourself! No one wants to look like they don't know the answer.

You must feel an urgency to have the answers to everything to become an efficient communicator. If you don't have the answers, people will not interact with you...they will simply say "Hello" in the beginning of their workout, and "Goodbye", when they leave. *You have to have interaction to be an effective communicator.* **(This is Teaching Anchor #3**).

Once you have a foot in the door and you've nailed that $8/hour job with your spray and towel in hand—befriend people. Walk around and learn people's names and ask them questions, such as:

"Why do you workout?"

"What do you do for a living?"

"What fitness goals do you have?"

"Where did you learn how to exercise?"

Listen to their comments and complaints. If they approach you about a specific concern, listen to them, and show them you have the power to rectify it. If you don't have the power or access to change it, tell them you will "***take care of it***". I guarantee they will begin to look at you in a different light if you follow up with their concerns. Begin to offer assistance. Don't be a seat warmer. Provide people with spots. Learn how to communicate non-verbally with others. Learn how to work together to get to a person's goal. Whether it is increasing someone's bench press or helping someone lose 15 pounds, you must learn what it is like to provide an **extension of yourself** to others. Most people classify themselves as good communicators simply because they are articulate when engaged in conversation. However, a good communicator does the engaging. Be an extrovert!

I have run into many personal trainers over the last 10 years, and I have to laugh at the ones that are self-gratifying. They think they are "so good" that whenever a client quits or doesn't reach their goal, it's not the trainer's fault—but the client is at fault. They tend to think that the client was lazy, unmotivated, un-focused, short-sighted, or just plainly fat. Most of these findings may be true, but what the trainer has failed to do is: <u>instruct, inspire, and integrate</u>. **(This is Teaching Anchor #4)**

Instruct – These are the practical skills you learn and what you teach. These are the tools from which your clients will build upon their success.

Inspire – Your empathy and attitude will help motivate clients to thirst for success.

Integrate – Develop a relationship with the client where you can have a direct effect on what outcomes he/she makes. Integrate yourself into the client's life.

Starting the Paper Process

Now let's start looking into getting some credentials. You should get your CPR certification to begin with. God forbid you will ever have to use this skill, but it is a perquisite to any personal training certification you plan to obtain. It is typically a 5-8 hour training course usually on a weekend or week night conducted at your local YMCA, local hospital, American Heart Association, or American Red Cross. Many other agencies also hold courses, including local community colleges, so begin to contact these sources and find out the dates.

You can check online for access to a CPR certification course at http://www.procpr.org/

Here's a quick assessment: If you don't desire to get your CPR certification because you don't want to sit in a room with a group of strangers and breathe into a dummy, or you feel it is a worthless skill to have because it has nothing to do with showing people how to exercise...<u>then forget personal training!</u> **(Remember Teaching Anchor #2...go back in the pages and re-read)** You need this qualification. Period.

Certifications

There are many reputable organizations that I can mention however; here are the ones that I have closely followed the last 10 years. In my opinion, there is an easy way to find out if a certification is worthy of attainment (and your hard-earned money): **the more difficult it is to get, the more weight [in the fitness industry] it carries.**

- **American College of Sports Medicine (ACSM)**
- **National Strength & Conditioning Association (NSCA)**
- **National Academy of Sports Medicine (NASM)**
- **National Endurance Sports Trainer Association (NESTA)**
- **American Council on Exercise (ACE)**
- **International Sports Sciences Association (ISSA)**

Here are a couple of scenarios you may encounter in your pursuit of a fitness certification:

Scenario #1.

If I go online to a search engine and input "personal training certification", I will get about 300 different organizations that certify. More than half of those certifications can be obtained simply by reading an online text and taking an online exam. ***Easy.***

Scenario #2

I can enroll in a personal training course at a local institution and have to attend classes, participate in practical hands-on work, and perform an internship to successfully pass the exam and become a fitness professional. ***Difficult.***

So the lesson of this particular content is that the easier you can earn a certification, the less reputation it may have in the industry.

If you don't already know, there are organizations that are collaborating to create one certifying body for personal training certifications and achieving national accreditation. So, it may become more exigent to obtain a reputable certification in the next 3-5 years.

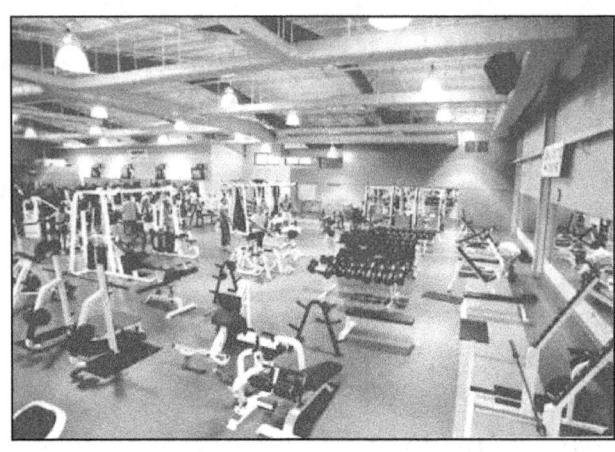

Hopefully, after 6-12 months you have obtained a piece of paper that says you passed a test to train others (certification). I would suggest you start looking at commercial fitness facilities for employment. You can stay at your organization or gym that you are currently employed; but unless you're in a facility that caters an environment for personal training needs and facilitating fitness goals, then I don't suspect you will grow [professionally] any more wiping down equipment and conducting orientations. Now I am suggesting you begin to think about throwing yourself into the pack of wolves...

The Wolves

Commercial facilities that strive on revenue growth and member retention usually stay abreast on fitness trends and like to dabble in what's new in the industry. This is to your advantage. You are not going to be the next VP of Bally's® or Gold's Gym®, but you will gain experience training a diverse clientele for a considerable compensation. Commercial facilities like to educate their staff in the latest fitness trends and will put out the cash for continuing education. The difference you will experience in a commercial facility like 24 Hour Fitness®, Ballys®, or Gold's Gym®, is the dependency on personal training for club revenues and overall profit. That is not entirely a bad thing. The more money your club makes, the more it can pay you. The more money made for the club, the more money can be allotted for continuing education on things like specialized certifications (if you decide to pursue specialized training in nutrition, sports, or older adult exercise).

Furthermore, the more it will spend on the latest strength equipment, which you will have the opportunity to use. However, this is all pending the mentality of the management. Ultimately, the more experience you get using the latest equipment and fitness tools, the more advanced you will be as a professional and have the flexibility to seek a higher compensation elsewhere.

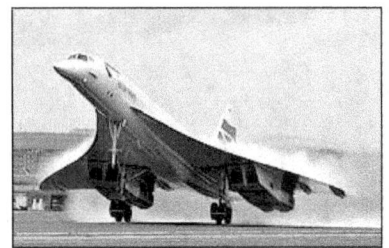

Remember the Concord Jetliner? Remember, it was so fast that it got passengers to their destination in a fraction of the time than a regular 747. It could fly from New York City to London in 2 hours! That's a typical 8 hour flight! Well, because Concord was so much more advanced among other commercial airlines, (and delivered on its promise), the company COULD ask for $5000 a ticket! Moral of that story? Appreciate the opportunities that are handed to you because they will give you experience and preparation for advancement. Once you are primed for advancement, your professionalism, experience, and skills are magnified reflecting an awesome resume that only demands a higher than normal salary!

Now, long gone are the days of sitting around and watching dust collect under the treadmills. In the pack of wolves, you have to be proactive and productive. That means selling your services.

Now when we think of selling, we think of 3 encounters:

- *Car salesman that sells you a junk automobile.*

- *Door-to-door salesman that tries to sell your mother a vacuum cleaner or set of encyclopedias.*

- *Cosmetic rep that cakes on as much make-up on your face, and then tries to sell you all of it.*

The common denominator among these salespeople mentioned is you can SEE what they are trying to sell you: car, appliance, furniture, make-up, house, etc. These are tangible items. In the world of personal training and fitness, prospective clients cannot see what you are trying to sell them which are **health and improved well-being**. They can imagine it, but most of the time, they have developed tough mental barriers [within themselves] that make the dream of a healthier body distant and unattainable.

In other words, it is challenging for the trainer to sell a package that costs $500 to a prospective client, and basically go on "promise" that you can get them there. Consumers like to see what they are paying for.

According to Steve Singleton, author of deeperstudy.com and a noted presenter, book editor, newspaper reporter, news editor, and public relations consultant, he has compiled a list of the "makes or Breaks of a Salesperson".

Professionalism
Professionalism also assumes well-honed organizational skills that make all contacts with the client a satisfying experience rather than an annoyance. What else distinguishes a professional from an amateur?

Commitment
If you are selling a product, your client expects you to be committed to delivering the highest value possible, as defined by their requirements. If you are selling a service, your client expects you to be as interested, even as passionate, about getting their job completed on time and on budget as they are themselves. Commitment to your company is also essential to your success, as

again and again you're current and potential clients ask you, "Why should I choose you over one of your competitors?" You must focus on providing a succinct but persuasive answer that question. Finally, you have to be committed to your own success-- committed enough to be highly disciplined in your investment of time, energy, training, and other resources to your own ongoing development. The committed keep growing.

Charisma

You may believe that personal magnetism is a gift you may or may not be born with, not a skill you can develop. Charisma, however, is a competence that all sales professionals need, and most are able to learn. It is that seamless combination of vision, empathy, self-confidence, enthusiasm, optimism, and focus that often makes the different between closing a sale and closing a door—right in your own face. It involves the consistent ability to rapport instantly and maintain it subconsciously so that you and your client are never adversarial, but on the same side. Yet if your charisma comes across as contrived or artificial, it will do more harm than good.

Work-ethic

Anyone who believes that success in sales is mainly good luck should remember the famous words of golfing great Lee Trevino, "It's amazing! The more I practice, the luckier I get." Developing and maintaining a good work ethic means that you develop efficient and effective work habits and then stick with them day in and day out. This includes a regular schedule, standard operating procedures for the repetitive tasks you must perform, a simple but effective record-keeping system, and the self-discipline to keep going no matter what. You recognize that your success is not dependent just on the number of hours you work, but on how much of that time you channel toward your objectives.

Desire

First; ask yourself, "What do I really want in my fitness career?" Once you have established a definite, satisfying, and enthusiasm-inducing answer, keep that goal at the forefront of your thinking all the time. Second, you must ask, "What do I really want for my client?" This second goal should remain your priority in your relationship with the client. That's what is known as "Customer Focus": meeting or exceeding the client's needs and expectations the first time and every time. The answers to these two questions should never be in conflict, but complementary. Desire is seldom a personality trait; so much as it is a developed skill. You think what you focus on, and you become what you think.

Attitude

As Zig Ziglar says, "It's your attitude, much more than you aptitude, that determines your altitude." Are you an optimist or a pessimist? Are you enthusiastic or lethargic? Do you look at the problems or the possibilities? Once more, contrary to those who say to themselves and to anyone else who will listen, "That's just the way I am," and "I can never seem to overcome this personality flaw I have," the right attitude is something we can develop, improve, and fine tune. Your mind will believe whatever you tell it about yourself. Why not choose to program it for success?

Creativity

If you are wondering what distinguishes you from one of your competitors, consider this: to the client you and other trainers may be indistinguishable; you may both be selling a superior product or service, and each of you may be delivering your presentation and maintaining contact in a truly professional manner. Your creativity might well become the sole differentiator that makes you stand out from the dozen cookie-cutter sales representatives your client has encountered. It may be a remarkable turn of phrase, a humorous leave behind, or an unforgettable story. What ever it is, creativity can easily become a factor between gaining an order and losing one. Creativity can be learned, developed, and enhanced.

Resilience

Anyone who has been in sales for very long has felt the pain of losing a close client. You may have invested many hours, days, or even weeks developing a relationship, gaining an opportunity to make a proposal, and earning your clients loyalty. Then the floor drops out, and you find the order has gone to a competitor or has been postponed indefinitely. Your ability on such occasions to bounce back not only to where you were before, but having gained from the experience, is one of the essential keys to sales success. If you are able to learn something from each loss and then put it behind you, your next opportunity has a higher likelihood for winning.

Flexibility

Every sales professional knows that success in selling is not simply a matter of following a checklist of do's and don'ts. You have to learn how to be flexible. In other words, you must develop an outstanding ability to read the particular needs, preferences, and personal idiosyncrasies of your client, and then tailor your interaction, presentation, and closing tactics to custom-fit that client. Employing a "one-size-fits-all," learned-by-rote sales system is one of the quickest ways you can find to convince your client that they don't matter to you.

Of course; each one of these has a rightful claim to your attention as important in and of itself. The challenge you face is to integrate all of these points into your personality as a fitness professional to the extent that they are convincingly natural. Only experience-- that is, recognizing and reinforcing your successful efforts while identifying and correcting your flops--can enable you to blend all of these characteristics into an outstanding sales persona that nevertheless is really you.

Empathy & Selling

There is one advantage that you have as a personal trainer over your average salesperson—you actually care about the other person! Hopefully, you do at least! A trainer gets into the business because they possess a passion for helping others---the identification with health, and the embodiment of leadership, coaching, and fitness combine into one role: fitness professional! A salesperson is motivated by commission!

What you also have is empathy. Empathy is consciously being aware of "where others have been" in certain circumstances or accidents. Empathy is not "feeling sorry", but having a sense of what perspires from a situation whether it is a death in the family, auto accident, failing a test, getting a speeding ticket, or being fat. How can this help you?

According to Jeff Blackwell, founder of salespractice.com, it is one of the simplest ways to be productive.

One of the simplest ways to increase your productivity as a personal trainer is to tune into your client's point of view. When you are in tune with your client you have empathy. This means that you can identify with and understand their situation, feelings, and motives.

When you are in tune with your client, everything you say or do seems to be right on the mark. The client gets the feeling that you really understand them and the road to a successful goal lights up like an airport runway. The opposite is also true. When you are not in tune with your client nothing you can do or say will seem to be right. When you push they pull and vice versa.

Master trainers know the importance of empathy and tune in to their clients as quickly as possible. Novice trainers on the other hand, rarely make the effort. This lack of empathy between client and trainer accounts for much of the negative experiences many gym-goers experience.

This kind of selling requires a genuine desire on the part of the personal trainer to try and be of service. It is pretty easy to spot the personal trainer with this kind of desire. These trainers take an interest in the client on a more personal level. The empathetic personal trainer asks more questions and better questions. They ask the type of questions that get the buyer to open up and talk about their situation.

Clients prefer a personal trainer that reaches them on a personal level. Everyone likes to be listened to and understood. Here are a few reminders to help you focus on your clients:

- **Focus your attention on your client. Do not allow yourself to become distracted.**

- **Look for something you like in the other person. What do you think their friends like about them?**

- **Get your client to tell you their situation, hopes and fears with well prepared questions.**

Sounds easy, right? Selling can be difficult for some people especially if your intent is to help as many souls as possible. I have run into many fitness professionals that favor the simple mantra of "improving the human spirit" out of passion and dedication of helping others. No problem, I

respect that. But if your intent is to help as many "souls" as possible---and make a living from it---then selling has to be a skill worth practicing. This is what I meant by the pack of wolves.

Hopefully, if you follow the foundation I laid out for you in the beginning chapters, you should develop a skill of creating rapport with strangers and building confidence and comfort in your professional skills. These characteristics and skills don't develop over night. Give yourself some time and reps talking to others. Hopefully, you are coming into this profession with a head-start by possessing some of the beneficial attributes mentioned.

The following pages contain a cut-to-the-chase table of favorable attributes to be a successful personal trainer. Take a look at them and score yourself honestly.

NO...don't pursue a career as a personal trainer if:

1.) If you get tired and bored in a stagnant gym setting.
2.) If you are impatient with people.
3.) If you don't have great organizational skills.
4.) If you do not possess the appropriate temperament.
5.) If you can't relate to different types of people.
6.) If you hate having different bosses. (In a sense, clients are your boss) **(This is Teaching Anchor #5)**
7.) If you don't like touching sweaty people.
8.) If you don't like invading another's space.
9.) If you can't be creative with exercise programming.
10.) If you can't talk about personal issues with clients.
11.) If you don't want to hear about clients' personal issues.
12.) If you are not a problem solver.
13.) If you don't like to supervise.
14.) Don't like inconsistent hours.
15.) Are not comfortable with your level of knowledge.
16.) If you cannot admit you don't have an answer.
17.) If you are not privy to change and new ideas.
18.) If you are selective with personalities.
19.) If you are more concerned with your look than your client's.
20.) If you can't look people in the eye.

YES...pursue a career as a personal trainer:

1.) If you can tolerate different levels of learning capabilities.
2.) If you find compassion discovering self-defeating behaviors in others.
3.) If you love watching people operate.
4.) Love dealing with different personalities in one day.
5.) Are a problem solver.
6.) Love to show others that you follow your own recommendations.
7.) Love making friends.
8.) Love seeing people become healthy and happy.
9.) If you are confident in your abilities.
10.) If you like having a flexible schedule.
11.) If you like learning new things.
12.) If you like advancement.
13.) If you become comfortable around strangers easily.
14.) Can be honest with yourself and strangers.
15.) Find joy in teaching exercises 8-10 times a day.
16.) Love to be creative.
17.) Can go the whole day without looking in the mirror.
18.) Can see multiple things going on at the same time.
19.) Can communicate non-verbally effectively.
20.) Can look people in the eye.

Have you figured out that many of the successes in being a personal trainer are based on your personality and communication skills? I haven't even started talking shop. This book is geared more towards helping you identify similarities between you and the role you want to play.

Teaching Anchors Explained

Throughout this book, you probably have seen bold-faced *"Teaching Anchors"* which are designed to distinguish key points that are important in the overall thought. If you missed them, shame on you. I advise you go back and look for them! Therefore, it is my responsibility to explain each anchor so that an understanding of each one can be developed. These are the true "secrets"...

Teaching Anchor #1:

"People that you share your company with become an extension of you."

Clients become your representatives. Not in the notion that they will make the sale for you, but in the fact that they represent everything you know. You service them in order to accomplish a goal. That goal is facilitated through your knowledge, expertise, and planning. If your client has attained a goal (fat loss, marathon completion, bigger bench, etc), then they accomplished it partially by what you taught them. They did this because every session, every set, and every rep you were there—encouraging, motivating, and understanding their struggle. Why do you understand their struggle? Because you represent this thing called fitness, and your goal is to **continuously** be a billboard of fitness (inside and outside the gym) for everyone to recognize. Maintaining this image becomes a kind of struggle for you.

Teaching Anchor #2

"You have to be in a position where you "service others".

Gas attendants pump your gas, waiters take your food order, and police officers protect you...so how do you service others in personal training? You have to understand and accept the position of helping others for the betterment of others, and not for self-serving pleasure. Help someone achieve their goal of fat loss because it is what they have struggled to do for years and with your help, they can actually accomplish it. Don't view these successes as notches under your belt, but rather, as more experience with the diversity of the human spirit. The human spirit can be strong or weak, sturdy or fragile, complicated or simple, driven or misguided. You "give" yourself to improve your own spirit.

Teaching Anchor #3

"You have to have interaction to be an effective communicator".

To be an effective communicator in personal training...and let me explain that: In order for your clients to perform the exercises you prescribe and execute them properly, you need to give them the instructions effectively. The difference between you and the newest issue of a muscle magazine is you can provide auditory, visual, and kinesthetic cues to your clients. A page in a magazine cannot. Remember: you can't communicate effectively if there is no interaction with the both of you. Sure, training one-on-one is a type of interaction, but not in the sense of being effective to convey your expertise. Usually, the clients you have really good relationships with are the ones that succeed. Why? Good communication not only provides effective instruction but also: support, rapport, openness, and caring.

Teaching Anchor #4

"Instruct...Inspire...Integrate."

This is not PhD material. This is stuff I realized through the years. This is the stuff that made me successful—successful in terms of the number of my clients that reached their goals—not how much money I made.

Instructing is the skills you acquire through education, experience, or certification courses. These are the skills that your exercise programming originates from.

Inspiring is the subconscious technique of putting into action the first three teaching anchors: realizing that clients are representative of you (extensions), servicing others, and being an effective communicator. These are the skills not taught in certification courses.

Integrating yourself into your client's life. I love trainers that start each sentence with, "I am going to have you do...", or 'I want you to perform...".

How about beginning each sentence: "WE are going to get to this by..." Do you see what I am talking about? <u>Good trainers make the client's goal—BOTH of their goals.</u>

Teaching Anchor #5

"The client is your boss."

Yes. It's true. Good trainers realize this. You work for every client. They don't work for you. Just as you can "fire" your client, they can also fire you. And if they fire you, it doesn't make you look good and you run the risk of bad-mouthing, loss of referrals, and loss of income. If you understand and apply the first 4 Teaching Anchors, then this last one should not be a problem. If you accept that every client is your responsibility and that you have goals (deadlines), and if you are insubordinate (tardy, habitual calling out, lying, etc), you can be let go! It is the trainers that don't believe this (or don't want to), they don't last more than 6 months in the business.

Show them they that you are a responsible professional from day one. Show them that you are respected among your peers and fellow staff. Show them that that you have accomplished a lot to earn their trust and business.

Shop Talk

The next few pages will detail some useful information that you, as a fitness professional, should be aware of when you actually begin transforming clients. Educating your clients will be the most important aspect of your job. I suggest you begin to "role-play" with friends, family, spouse, or co-workers. Being a problem solver is important as a personal trainer as you will fight against a host of deterrents including:

- ☐ **Self-defeating behaviors**
- ☐ **"Gym science"**
- ☐ **Quick fix marketing**
- ☐ **Ignorance to exercise**
- ☐ **Unsupportive client spouses**
- ☐ **Client time management**

The first thing you should acclimate yourself with are the benefits of physical activity: moving. Since over half of the American population is overweight, 95% of your clients will share the same fitness goal of fat loss. Calorie expenditure is important for health for many reasons. The first thing you see when you walk into a fitness center is treadmills, ellipticals, and bikes. Remember when you used to clean them? Remember when you heard the hum of the treadmills all day? Well, now we are going to use them.

Understanding Cardio for Your Clients

If you're a weight-training enthusiast, no doubt you know the benefits to be gained from building strong muscles. But, is cardio training part of your workout, too? If it's not, you should consider adding it to your routine. Weight training paired with cardiovascular workouts provides a nearly perfect combination for keeping you fit and healthy. Let's look at seven reasons to add cardio training to your workout.

Cardio Training is Good for Your Heart - The increased heart rate you will achieve during your cardio workout will improve the condition of your heart and lungs, by training your heart to pump more blood in fewer beats and your lungs to move more oxygen with less effort. The improvement you will gain in your cardiovascular health will reduce your risk of heart disease and improve your blood cholesterol and triglyceride levels. Aim for 30-60 minutes at least 3 days a week in order to achieve the best results for improving your heart.

Cardio Training Will Help Improve Muscle Mass - Yes, it's true - You need strength training to gain muscle, but the thirty minutes you spend on those elliptical trainers will help improve your muscle mass, too, especially if you combine the two as part of an interval training program. By going back and forth between cardio training and weight training, you are working your muscles and then letting them relax several times during a workout, which will improve your ability to build that great toned look. In addition, regular aerobic exercise causes the capillaries in your muscles to grow, which helps them to remove waste, such as lactic acid, from your body more easily. This will help improve the health of your muscles, and reduce muscle soreness after your workout.

Cardio Training Burns Fat - Adding four thirty minute cardio sessions a week to your current training schedule will help you rev up your fat burning capability. The fat loss you will see will help your toned muscles be even more noticeable.

Cardio Training Revs Up Your Metabolism - In addition to the fat you will burn during your workout, regular cardiovascular training will boost your metabolism for hours after your workout, too, helping you to maximize fat loss all day long.

Your Immune System Can Improve - People who spend thirty minutes in cardiovascular exercise at least three times a week are less likely to catch colds and other viral illnesses. It is believed that aerobic exercise improves your immune system, making it better able to fight off infection.

Your Mental State Will Improve - Cardio training causes your brain to release endorphins, the body's natural high. Endorphins act as natural painkillers and stress reducers.

You Are Likely To Live Longer - The New England Journal of Medicine has found a direct link between regular exercise and longevity.

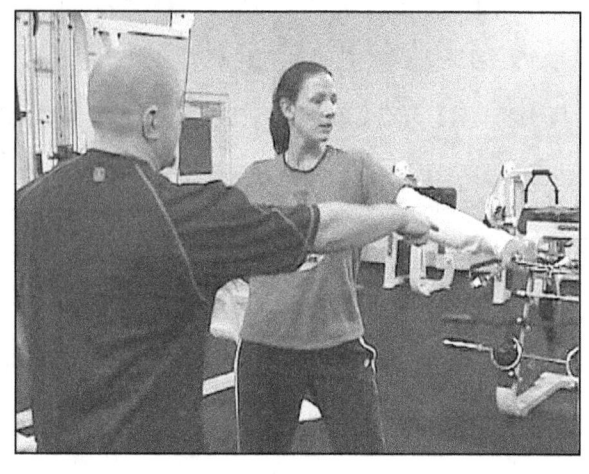

Exercises That Should Be Taught

I am often confused when I see seasoned personal trainers acquire new clients and begin their exercise program with some strength training circuit or group exercise class. I often wonder what is the trainer thinking when they are devising this person's exercise program? Were they thinking at all? I know 95% of client goals are based on fat loss and very few choose "be athletic". But do you know how many times I have told clients, *"You don't want to be an athlete, but you want to look like one?"*

So the wheels begin to turn and the education process begins. The physique of an athlete reflects the protocol of performance training. Athletes have been shown to be more in-tune with muscular control, alertness, proprioception, elasticity, and power...not to mention higher levels of lean body mass and decreased body fat.

So what do you do with a general population client (GPC)? The main objective of a fitness professional should be to improve function. No matter what the goal is. A competent trainer will understand that by improving function and performance, you will elicit muscle gain and fat loss. If the trainer does not understand that, he or she must go back to their textbooks and read again. So what kind of performance training does the GPC need? They need performance enhancement of activities of daily living (ADLs). GPC's are typically made up of homemakers, business people, weekend warriors, marathon runners, or active older adults. However, the main performance improvement training (PIT) protocol begins with mastering progressions of primal movements.

An efficient human body *(meaning one without congenital functional restrictions or history of injury, surgery, or mental trauma)* should be able to perform five basic primal movements learned within the first 4 years of life. The 5 basic functions of human performance translated into exercise are:

1.) **Squat**
2.) **Lunge**
3.) **Step-Up**
4.) **Push-up**
5.) **Ab Crunch**

These basic exercises are precursors to numerous loaded and unloaded exercises. The job of a personal trainer is to get the client as close to flawless with these 5 movements as possible. You don't have to get them to EXACTLY 100% flawlessness, but awfully close. How close? **Absolutely no GPC should progress to**

any other advanced movement until body control skills have improved, "fundamental strength" has increased, and pain/discomfort has vanished. How long will this take? Just like any other exercise program adherence, the timeline to performance improvement in these exercises depends on client/trainer interaction, frequency, proper cueing, and effective instruction. I have seen clients improve on these 5 exercises in 1 week, and some 3-4 weeks. The wonderful thing about beginning any exercise program with these primal movement exercises is that any discussed or fathomed pains ("my knee has problems when I climb stairs" or "my shoulder aches in the morning upon waking") *seem to disappear.*

Most of today's movement assessments are based around these five exercises. For the trained fitness professional, they can serve as analytical information regarding muscle imbalances, weakness, tightness, dysfunction, history of injury, and baseline testing procedures. Another advantage to developing exercise programs around these 5 exercises is there is no need for equipment or space. Clients can work on these primal movements in the convenience of their homes, hotels, or park. Remember, one of the factors I discussed earlier in regards to timeline of progression was frequency. How often are they performing these five exercises correctly on their own? And if the instruction and cueing is potent, advanced movements can be added leading to faster results.

Squat

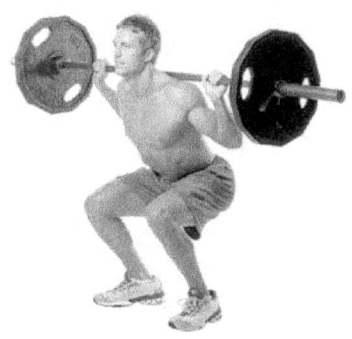

The squat is performed in most sporting situations. However, it is also performed by GPC with every visit to the lavatory. You laugh, but this is why these 5 exercises are deemed "primal". The human body should be able to perform these exercises if there is no congenital defect, function altering injury, or neurological impedance. The squat exercise involves bilateral, symmetrical, and functional mobility of the hips, knees, and ankles. The ability to perform the squat correctly requires appropriate pelvic rhythm, closed-chain dorsiflexion of the ankles, flexion of the knees and hips, and extension of the thoracic spine.

Lunge

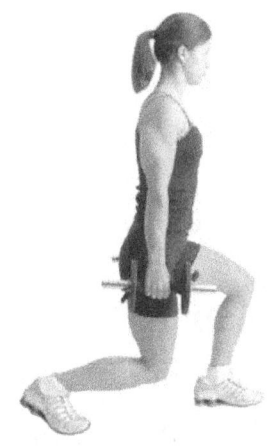

The lunge is another primal movement that puts the body in a position that will focus on the stresses as simulated during rotational, decelerating, and lateral movements. The lunge places the lower body in a "scissored" position—similar to walking, jogging, and running—and requires stability in the stance leg (ankle, knee and hip) and closed chain hip abduction. The difficulty with the lunge in GPC's is the lack of stability due to the rotational stress imposed. Bottom line...master the lunge and you are on your way to improve your walking and running mechanics.

Step-up

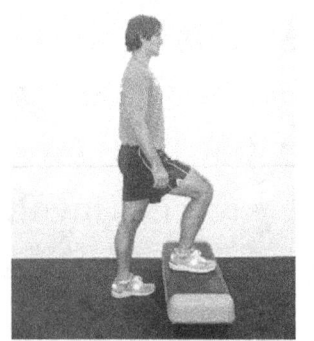

Another primal movement that simulates activities of daily living (walking up and down stairs, overcoming curbs, getting in and out of a car) is the step-up. The step up helps in challenging the body's stride mechanics using proper coordination and stability between the hips and torso. The step up is perfect for assessing bilateral function mobility and stability of the hips, knees, and ankles. In addition, the step-up exercise also involves adequate balance because of the demand for dynamic stability.

Push-up

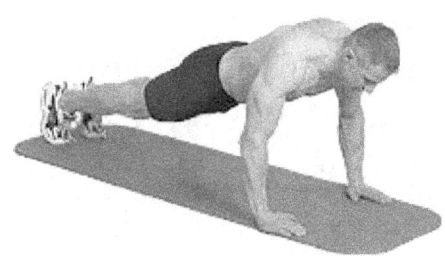

This upper body closed chain exercise is the single best primal movement for upper body performance improvement. The push-up stresses trunk stability in the sagital plane. Many activities require the trunk stabilizers to transfer force symmetrically from the upper extremities to the lower extremities and vice versa. If the trunk lacks stability, energy will disperse leading to poor functional performance, and increased chance of chronic injury. I have always been a fan of teaching clients the same cue's I instruct them with, so that when they perform these exercises alone, they can visualize that correct positioning that I would request. One deviation from what I desire in a push-up is the *"clothesline-effect"*. This is characterized by the client getting into a standard push-up position and performing 2-3 reps before witnessing the neck jut forward, and the abdominals fall down as if they are leading the exercise with the mid-section. In the same manner as a clothesline that has too many wet clothes in the center and both ends are stable. The "straight line" disappears. We want to maintain that line beginning with the trunk. Ideally, all GPC should begin this exercise in the modified position with knees on floor and ankles crossed. To decrease the lever arm (in this case, the trunk) allows the client more muscular control and proper execution of cues. Once the modified version is acceptable, the standard position can commence.

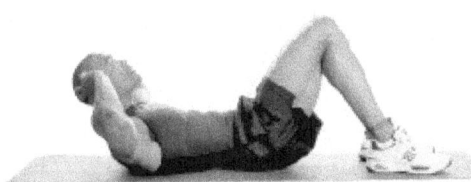

Crunch

How many times are you going to be on your back and perform spinal flexion? Every morning you do. Unless you are a bat and hang upside-down. The crunch gets a lot of flack because it has been regarded as *non-functional* to sport and is merely a cosmetic exercise. However, if properly cued, the ab crunch can help the GPC engage the abdominals while accentuating proper TVA firing. *Ahh...the beginnings of core work.* Think about it...every morning you get up from a 7-8 hour sleep without a warm-up and rotate your trunk. I used to have clients perform a simple task of laying supine on the floor and practicing getting up. After they would get up, they would lie back down and repeat 10-15 times! Movement times decreased in the first week. Clients got up faster and had more control. Talk about functionality!

Personal Trainer Validity

With the abundance of new personal trainers entering the field every year (by the way, that's 25,000 new trainers entering the field every year), and the popularity of personal training through shows like "Biggest Loser®", the public can become smarter when shopping around for your services.

A great article by David Peterson of BOSS Fitness (www.bossfitness.com) examines the validity of personal trainers and a few cues prospective clients can use to spot good trainers from bad trainers. Read on...

Is your personal trainer qualified? How experienced are they? How can you know before committing to a long-term agreement? These are all questions that clients looking to hire a personal trainer have or should have.

Personal trainers hold a great deal of responsibility in their hands, as they "direct" their clients how to exercise safely and effectively. Personal training can be a lucrative career too, with some trainers charging as much if not more than doctor or lawyer consultation rates.

It is unlikely that you would hire a lawyer or a doctor strictly on hearsay, popularity, or if they "looked the role" but rather you would spend a good deal of time researching his or her credentials, track record, and education. So if you are going to pay a personal trainer equivalent fees ($100-$300/hour), shouldn't choosing an exercise professional be any different?

Rather than re-hash the details of the typical "How to Choose a Personal Trainer" cliché, this article provides the lay consumer just two helpful pieces of information to help when deciding on how to choose a personal trainer.

Grading a Trainer's Qualifications

A personal trainer is an exercise professional so their credentials should demonstrate this. Check to see if the trainer has had a formal education in exercise science, physiology or sports medicine.

Exercise is about science and is grounded firmly in the fields of anatomy, physiology and nutrition. Each field complements and builds on the other. Even the most experienced (or well-built!) personal trainer cannot fake knowledge he does not have. A thorough understanding of these fields is essential to effective and safe exercise instruction and is unlikely to be gained in a weekend or even a multiple week study course.

The client looking to hire a personal trainer should also check the certifying organization. Currently the most respected credentials are offered by the NSCA (National Strength and Conditioning Association), NASM (National Academy of Sports Medicine), ACSM (American College of Sports Medicine) and ACE (American Council on Exercise).

Some certifying bodies such the NSCA require certain educational requirements to be completed before sitting for the exam. An example is the NSCA's Certified Strength and Conditioning Specialist (CSCS), which requires a bachelor's degree in a related field to sit for the exam.

Grading a Trainer's Experience

An experienced and well-educated exercise professional can easily recognize others on par with themselves simply by observing the manner in how they work with their client and by watching the client's exercise technique.

What about the casual exerciser who knows nothing of exercise or fitness? How can they discern the small details that give clues to a trainer's experience and quality of instruction? After all, certification only means that the personal trainer passed a written exam.

The answer is that it is very tricky for a layperson to judge personal trainers themselves from simple observation and as a result, may rely too heavily on the opinion of others.

Don't get me wrong there is nothing more valuable to a personal trainer than a good reputation and "word of mouth", but an informed consumer looking for a quality exercise professional should do a little more homework.

While there may be dozens of time consuming and complicated ways to assess a personal trainer's instruction quality and experience, this article describes a single test that will give the client a basic insight before committing to a contract or agreement. A client should not be embarrassed or scared to use this test; it is the full right and privilege of the client to interview and consult with the trainer before committing on a long-term or contractual basis.

Retaining Clients – Part 1

Once you have achieved some success in personal training by acquiring clients and helping them change physically through your awesome exercise programming and motivation, you need to begin to think how to keep them coming when they are beginning to feel they don't need you anymore.

I believe that in order for a trainer to call him/her "successful", we must examine his/hers' ability to "keep" current clients. In the field of personal training, where motivation and personality are as vital as practical knowledge, the mainstay of those attributes lies in the ability for a client to reach their fitness goal. Obviously, if a client reaches a fitness goal, they will thank you and flourish you with an abundance of praises. With those accolades come great marketability, referrals, and increased confidence levels. With confidence comes a map to success. Once you taste success, you want to experience it **every time**.

However, there are bumps along the way. A busy trainer doesn't just have one client or maybe two. A busy trainer usually has 20 and up to 45 clients per week. Trying to motivate all your clients on a weekly basis can be a tedious, energy consuming skill. So I understand that sometimes when you are down to your sixth or seventh client of the day, you are tired, drained, and hungry. People like you and me wake up every morning "planning" to attend the gym or exercise. Sedentary individuals that have entered the "action" stage need constant accountability and *motivation to adhere to a plan*. This can be difficult for the trainer, so I understand that you don't always keep every client you obtain. You do get "drop-outs" and that is normal in the personal training field.

I also understand that for every lost client you suffer (as a trainer); you must try to obtain two or three new ones. In order to make a living at personal training and enjoy it as a profession, it needs to be rewarding on a human level and financial level. This means preparing for client drop-outs.

Many trainers that begin in the field start out with a passion to help others—which is the main foundation of the craft—but then they realize that they have to work at retaining regular clients. They begin to hate the "business" side of personal training. They hate the "work" aspect of the career. That is fine too. I don't think there is a company in the world that employs staff with an equal level of work production. Some employees go above and beyond because they are motivated by one thing and some remain satisfactory because they are motivated by other things. The differences are seen in their salaries, stature, and attitude.

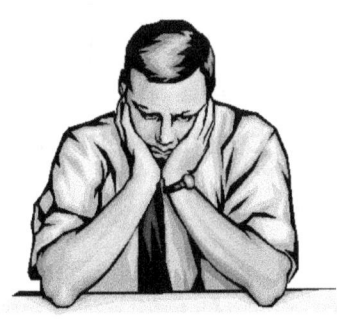 So what does this have to do with anything? I'll tell you a story about a friend of mine. He is a great guy and is a personal trainer. He loves sharing his knowledge with people and is quite good at it. However, he is unhappy with the fact that he is only paid based on the amount of work he puts into drumming up his business. For instance: he can only "handle" 5 clients a week at $70 a session each. That's only $350 a week he is earning for his services. He doesn't want to look for prospective clients because it takes a lot of effort to build new rapport; design a new exercise program; assess; and carry out that plan; so his business suffers and so does his wallet. His clients experience his frustration with the direction his career is going and sense a loss of passion on his part. This can be experienced by monotony in workouts, decreased energy and enthusiasm during sessions, and frequently

cancelled sessions (by both parties). So my friend would rather rely on **passive** income. Well, once he begins to rely on passive income, he realizes that passive income is sporadic and is not constant like **active** income. Active income requires constant attention and drive. Active income requires that you get up every morning and try your hardest to lure in a new client to replace the clients you will eventually lose. Active income resembles the time you spend developing an ongoing exercise program for a client....all the research you do for a client...all the templates you put together for a client....and all the openness you share with a client. But in the end, my friend just sits back down and is satisfied with his $350 a week.

Good trainers will always have clients that have been with them for years. And you know who these clients are? They fall into 2 categories:

a.) Clients who experience success (have lost fat or gained muscle) or
b.) Clients whom love the interaction and camaraderie with a personal trainer.

With either category, the trainer is enjoying a continuous flow of income AND constant referral source. Clients that stay with you for long periods are your best marketers. They talk about your workouts, your personality, your work ethic, your passion, and your commitment to help them achieve their goals. With so much admiration being created for you as a personal trainer, why wouldn't anyone want to work with you?

So if you are presently a personal trainer--on your own or through a health club---here are 5 tips to help you retain your clients or get new ones:

1.)   Always use the term "We".
In your communication with your client, always use the term "we".

"We will get to your goal in 6 weeks"...
"We ought to be able to hit that 225 bench next week"...
"We better get to it because your marathon is coming up".

Clients love feeling like they are in a partnership with you. Clients look up to the personal trainer and when they feel like you are "sharing" their fitness goal, they feel more supported, more confident, and more obligated to not let you [personal trainer] down.

2.)   Show the client the right <u>and</u> wrong way to perform an exercise.
I have always demonstrated the right way and wrong way of an exercise to a client because I believe it empowers the client with knowledge. I believe that if a client can visually see the wrong way to perform an exercise, they are more likely to

perform it correctly. I even go so far as point out people in the gym performing exercises incorrectly to my client. And while we stand there and watch, I'll explain "why" and "what exactly" is wrong with the way the exercise is being performed. This act of empowerment builds trust between you and the client, and also, confirms your role as the educator.

3.) Don't be afraid to speak to your client about things other than exercise!

I see this all the time. The trainer and client are finished with a set and they just stand there and don't say two words to each other. There is no communication! The trainer must not be afraid to talk about the weekend; or the kids; or the TV show they watched last night—**just don't get lost in the conversation!** How awkward is it for the client who grunts and sweats in front of their trainer every day, but does not feel comfortable around them? You must establish a relationship with your client, and it is okay to talk about life with them. It's okay to cross that line minimally. So many trainers are robots and become fearful of "being unprofessional". But guess what? YOU control what you say. YOU control what you talk about. YOU control how long you want to talk. This leads me to number four.

4.) The trainer must control the session.

A client must understand that the fitness professional must steer the session. Some clients may be CEO's or aggressive types, but in the fitness realm—you are the CEO! If you are confident in your ability, confident in YOUR workplace, and you are confident that you can help your client—then you must control the session. You must control the exercise selection, the pace, conversation length, and rest periods. The trainer has "home-field advantage" and needs to establish the direction and leadership.

5.)   Acknowledge your other clients when you see them
Let's say you are in the middle of a training session with your client, Jane. As you are training Jane, you see your other client Bob. You and Bob usually work on Tuesdays and today is Friday. As you keep your eyes on Jane performing single leg hip bridges, you acknowledge Bob with a head nod and a smile. The simple act of assuring him that you have noticed he's made an effort to come in for a workout on his own can do wonders for your client. Even the ones you are not currently with! I can't tell you how many times---and how bright a client's face lit up---when I would recognize him/her by name whenever I was working with another client. As people, we all like to be acknowledged by name or face. So, don't have blinders on with one client....keep your eyes moving across the entire gym floor and "scan" for your regulars. These traits are what score you the next potential new client. And I guarantee, if you apply these 5 tips to your present client list....you should have an easy time receiving referrals or obtaining the woman on the

treadmill that watched you every morning train your 10 o'clock client!

Retaining Clients – Part 2

So now that we have covered the role and characteristics of a personal trainer; the expectations for success in the business of personal training; and the level of skill needed, we will now explore more methods of retaining your clients. Why? Retaining your clients will assure you of the following:

- **Continuous income**
- **Constant experience in progressive exercise programming**
- **Constant experience in communication skills.**
- **Possible future referrals.**
- **Greater chances of client success because you will spend more time with them.**
- **Great reputation.**

You will always have a few clients that are your favorites. These are the ones that you feel closest to and can be very personable with.

So what do you do to try to keep them? Become their friend but keep your professional distance. Yes, it is possible. As a fitness professional, you fall into the same category as doctors and lawyers do with their relationships with patients and clients, respectively. That means dealing with concerns of confidentiality and trust. Once the session is over or the client stops training with you, you must maintain a level of professionalism which means keeping personal information, discussions, and records confidential.

You should also ask your clients for honest criticism. There is no other effective way of finding out how you are doing as a trainer, than by asking your client about your sessions, demeanor, attitude, and exercise program.

Your client's feedback can be the difference between improving your business and losing it right away; knowing where you succeed and where you fail is critical to growing your business and achieving success in the field. The best way to get that feedback is by sending surveys to your clients asking questions like:

- *How has my service worked for you?*
- *In what ways do you think I can improve my service?*
- *In which areas do you think I could improve my communication skills?*
- *From one to ten, how many points would you give me for "listening to you"?*
- *Would you recommend me to your friends?*
- *Can you shortly describe your experience with me?*

Deeply analyze the answers you get from your clients. Those answers are gold for you, because they provide valuable opinions from your clients you won't be able to have otherwise. It may sound crazy, but we often don't make suggestions if people don't ask us first, and when they do, a feeling of importance may make us invest the proper time to give the most detailed, sincere suggestions we can think of.

How much would you pay to know where you succeed and where you fail in your business? It's priceless to have that kind of information at your disposal just by picking up the phone or sending an email to one of your beloved clients. While hiring a consultant or sending an employee to grab some feedback from your clients about your product or service can be very tempting, it may not have the same outcome as doing it yourself! (They are taking the time to answer your questions after all; why send someone else to make them or to pick up the answers?)

Keeping "You" In "Their" Minds

An easy way to sell is through your existing clients; that's a fact. If you can keep yourself on your client's minds long enough every several weeks, they will keep buying from you or they will send you some referrals for you to work with—which is even better. As a fitness professional, you should drop clients an e-mail now and then; or make a phone call to acknowledge their workout program. Try to keep them focused on the goal. During holiday season, drop them a card or bake them a healthy snack!

Direct mail or newsletter work pretty well in this department too, but there is no replacement for client's feedback because you will not only get first-hand information about what you're doing right and wrong with your business and how you may improve those aspects, but you will also be putting yourself in your client's mind, and that will lead into new contracts and contacts.

Conclusion

So hopefully after reading this book you have an understanding that being a successful personal trainer and being recognized as such, is more or less about having great people-skills. You don't have to have the type of skills that put you in front of a podium and speak to hundreds of people—although someday they may get you there; and you don't have to have the type of skills that help run a country—although they may get you there too. In the end, you have to serve your clients and remember that they are a **representative of you**. Your client represents your passion, your knowledge, your skills, and your commitment to the betterment of others through fitness.

I hope that this book has given you insight and clearer view of the world of helping others. Be it athletes, older adults, youth, or baby boomers, all can be *saved* through exercise. And as "physician extenders", you will be doing your part in the realm of preventative medicine...all through your love of fitness.

The following pages contain articles written by the author. These articles have been previously published on various fitness websites and have proven to be very helpful.

Secret Skills of Personal Training
Articles

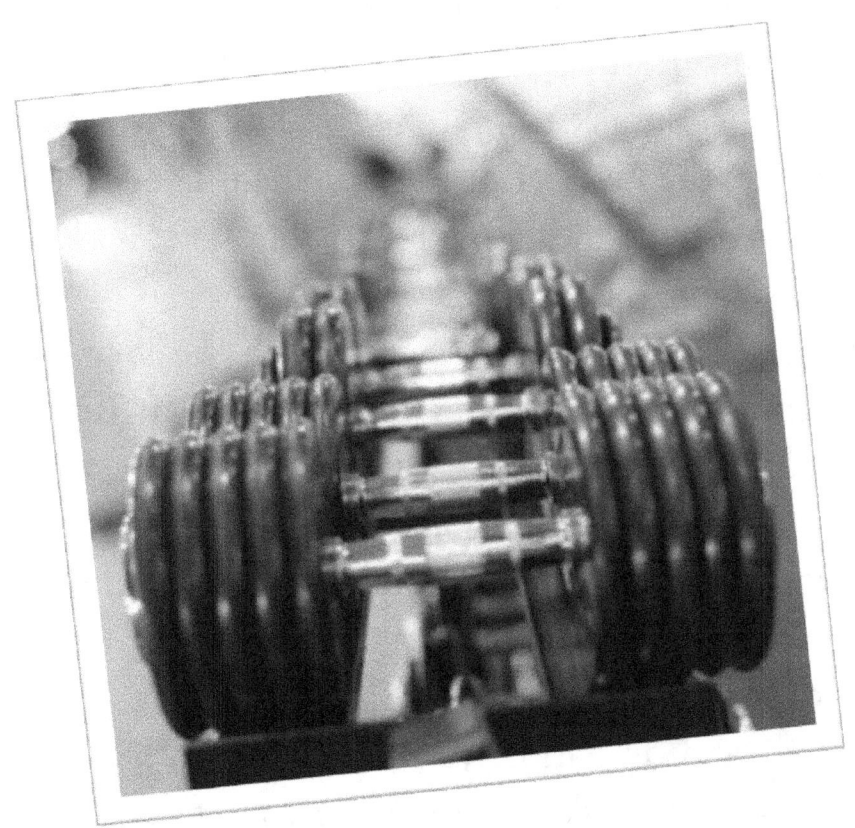

Personal Trainer Prerequisites
10 Tasks Every Trainer Should Be Able to Perform
By John Izzo

Real simple...if you want to be respected by your peers and gain notoriety amongst colleagues, fellow staff, or your bosses, then you should be proficient at these 10 tasks. Although it is not the "end all, be all" list of tasks that define you as a person, they do set a benchmark for the level of professionalism needed to solidify a status as a professional fitness trainer.

How was this list compiled? Easy...through the years I have had the opportunity to interview over 50 trainers at the 3 different facilities I have managed. Some I have hired, most I have never called or seen again. Some of these traits were easily identifiable in interviewees and some needed some fostering and instruction. Nonetheless, those trainers went on to experience some success in the field. Some of the tasks are not going to be completed before you enter the field or within your first year. Some of the tasks reflect your character and how it correlates to the field of personal training (i.e. dealing with client issues), while others reflect your understanding and preservation of academia and concepts learned through the process. However, you should concentrate on working towards proficient completion of each one within 2 years in the field. Each task will ensure you become capable and skillful as a fitness professional to your peers, your clients, and most importantly...yourself.

All Good Trainers Should...

...be multi-tasked. Trainers have an enjoyable job that lets their passion lead them, but there is always the need to be organized and professional. The ability to schedule appointments, prepare ahead of time, and return phone calls—all at the same time—is the grain of this profession. The more aptitude you demonstrate, the more likely you are to maintain a consistent schedule and reap the rewards of word of mouth business and successful planning.

...have an assertive personality. I usually tell new trainers that if they are not a "people person", then they are in the wrong field. Half of this profession is filled with educated trainers that can design an entire off-season program for a dozen lacrosse players—but have the personality of bird-cage paper. Education is an important element to have in this field, but without the proper vehicle (personality) to convey that knowledge, it makes it virtually handicap to the receiver. The ability to converse with your clients abuts off-topic issues and maintains their focus on the exercise at hand is critical and a very important "middle-ground" to have when sustaining a profitable client load.

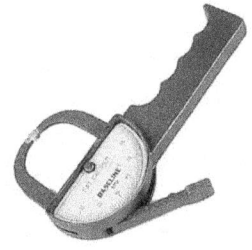 **...perform skin-fold (caliper) measurements.** I know the use of the bio-impendence analyzer (Omron) is popular and easy to use; however, it is still not as accurate as a properly performed skin-fold test. This simple fact is enough reason for all

trainers to take the responsibility to become proficient at using the Lange® or Skyndex® caliper. Since the introduction of the Omron to the market and mainstream fitness, most new trainers forego the task of performing caliper testing as an alternative to body fat measuring. This is an error. Learning and becoming efficient at using calipers projects an image of professionalism and skill. Most detractors will argue that clients feel intimidated and uncomfortable with even the sight of a Lange caliper; however, with the proper instruction and explanation, a trainer can perform the body fat assessment with a caliper—even on the opposite gender. Most 3, 4, and 7 site tests include simply lifting or adjusting clothing—but never fully removing. I understand that you may still have clients that feel uncomfortable with this, but with proper explanation and professionalism, a client should feel comfortable enough to "give" themselves to you during this 1 minute test.

...name at least 3 top fitness experts or their work (which you've hopefully read). It disheartens me when I have a conversation with some trainers, who have been in the field for a number of years, and they do not recall any of the sources that I cite in my programs or articles. For instance, by now you should know who Michael Boyle, Stuart McGill, Juan Carlos Santana, or Alwyn Cosgrove is. You should know or have read some of the written materials that they have produced to help reassure that your programming is up to date. Books like "Functional Training for Sports", "Athletic Body in Balance", "Low Back Disorders",

"Starting Strength", and "Diagnosis and Treatment of Movement Impairment Syndromes" should be on your "to read" list. Among the hundreds of resources available today, it is important to continue the learning process from those that are more learned that you. The internet has enabled users to obtain information from millions of resources across the world—albeit the more important it becomes to make sure that the resources your do acquire your additional information come from reliable and trusted sources. Here are a couple of good websites that are worthy of your valuable time to gain more info:

http://www.ptonthenet.com/default.aspx;
http://www.physsportsmed.com/,
http://www.training-conditioning.com/

...maintain a <u>minimum</u> client load of 10-12 sessions per week. I know, it doesn't seem like much, but it ensures that you are serious about this career. Keeping a dozen people happy is harder than keeping 3 people happy and easier than keeping 25 happy. So 12 is a well-rounded goal to meet for a minimum. Most trainers that work part-time typically stay in the field "part-time". Trainers who dabble with fewer client hours or typically work another 40-hour week job (not fitness related) tend to not fully grasp the on-going learning process; lack program creativity; and tend to miss client sessions or be tardy at them. If you are currently under 10-12 hours per week in actual training sessions and you are content with that amount, my advice would be to challenge yourself to learn a new concepts and take your continuing education seriously.

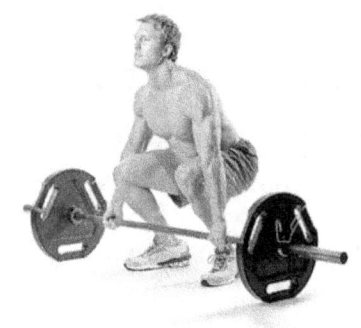

...be able to properly instruct a client to perform the Squat, Deadlift, & Push-up.
Over the years, nothing has been more and more compelling to me than the importance of these three movements. It wasn't until I really understood why they were important that they became staples in every one of my clients' programs. When you have a comprehension of human biomechanics and real-life functionality—the role of the squat, deadlift and push-up become clear. These movements help improve the body's natural locomotive mechanism and assist in the progression of external loading. These movements are translated in everyday life and more often than not, are tattered with poor compensatory patterns and dysfunction. The typical general population client picks his briefcase up every day poorly; or has trouble standing from a seated position; or the simple task of closing a door becomes cumbersome because the over-abundance of joint deficiencies have caused these primal movement patterns to be lost through age, inactivity, atrophy, and injury. The simple, yet effective instruction , of these three exercises can propel a trainer to success—yet, too many trainers view this task as either "too simple and not overly complicated" so it is skipped in exercise programming for balance and "core work"; or they are not proficient enough themselves in

performing them. In either case, if you are a trainer who is not sure how to perform these three movements, I suggest you hire yourself a good fitness trainer and learn them.

...be able to improvise. The ability to make acute changes in daily programming and exercise approach are key elements in showing a client that the trainer is able to lead. Many trainers lose focus and grasp when an unforeseen situation presents itself during a session. For example, if a client is trained in a commercial facility that boasts a large amount of people in attendance, chances are space and exercise selection may be limited—even though, the trainer has a sequence in mind to use with the client. If the trainer can make subtle changes during the session –without the client's acknowledgment-- then the trainer has kept the client's focus, trust, and confidence intact. If you have these three fundamental traits covered, you are sure to have a successful client.

...be flexible. I am not speaking in terms of free time; I am talking about physically having a heightened degree of flexibility. Trainers should be able to demonstrate flexibility exercises with ease and precision. I am not speaking that you should be able to perform a "split" or be a yoga queen, but I think trainers should be able to demonstrate active hamstring stretches, piriformis stretch, self-myo-fascia release, and similar exercises without a hitch. Clients are more inclined to stretch on a regular basis if they are taken through the flexibility exercises with the trainer during each session. This also ensures clients will remember how to perform the stretch correctly if they can "see" it performed by you.

...be able to tell the client WHY he/she is performing a particular exercise. Many new trainers tend to "memorize" exercises or seek out only the photos in books, magazines, or websites. There is no problem with learning new exercises, movements, and drills to share with your client or class; however, the trainer should understand the following for each new exercise learned and prior to having a client perform:

- *What muscles is the exercise using?*
- *What plane of motion does this exercise utilize?*
- *What joint actions are occurring?*
- *What type of load (if any) is appropriate with this exercise and is it conducive to the client's goal?*
- *Is the exercise efficient as a primary movement or as an auxiliary exercise?*

I should also note that the trainer should perform a new exercise a number of times on oneself before administering it to a client. The trainer should be able to spot any deviations from perfect form and find biomechanical cues to instruct to the client.

Here are some good resources to learn more about the "how's" and "why's" of exercise:

http://www.getbodysmart.com/

http://www.rad.washington.edu/academics/academic-sections/msk/muscle-atlas

http://www.performanceworkouts.com/exercise_guides_full_1.shtml

http://www.physicalfitnet.com/

...be able to perform a single leg exercise. Trainers know that the importance of single leg work translates to improved functionality for the general population client; and the regular use of single leg work attributes to improved proprioceptive communication between the ground and foot, then why can't many fitness trainers accomplish a single leg squat? Please don't let this prerequisite scare you into thinking you should become a "pistol" squatting fool, but it should make you aware that if you, as a trainer, practice what you preach and understand the importance of single leg work—not as a circus act, but as a component of a sound exercise program—whether for athlete or grandmother—then the conversion of this training into real-life activities makes the trainer more effective for his/her client.

Why 50% of Personal Trainers Suck
By John Izzo

So, being labeled a personal trainer has come around over the last 3-4 years. Being one is not as foreign as it used to be when I first started out. Of course, they're those that started out before me. Oh, yeah...they were called Biff, Zach, and Lance. They were the biggest guys in the gym with the darkest tans, and the highest Ottomix® shoes around. They wore bandanas, belts, and earrings in the gym. They smelled like protein and they had more weightlifting gloves than some women had shoes. Some were old too...frequently telling me stories of feats past—big benches, big deads, big squats....torn pecks, bad backs, and messed up knees.

So these guys eventually fizzled out and a new breed of trainers came around. These trainers came out of college with degrees and athletic backgrounds. These new trainers came out of aerobics rooms and sought out certifications. These new trainers rose up out of the dungy gyms and became students of the game. These new trainers used what they learned in books and did research on themselves. They understood the function of the hamstring in a lunge is to decelerate the movement....they understood the function of the rotator cuff...they understood that cardiovascular performance was directly related to functional capacity. These new trainers even looked professional. They wore khaki's, polo and golf shirts, dress shoes, and had smiles. These new trainers practiced what they preached because they learned in their own trainings; they learned in athletics; they learned in step classes; and they learned through trial and error. These trainers had a passion to share the knowledge they obtained with the average joe and once they were able to help their first client...*a confidence was born*. These trainers understood that their passion was becoming their bread and butter. These trainers began to understand selling their services was part of the game and they wanted to market their success to more and more clients. They understood they can achieve longevity in this field, rather which assuming it was a short term career detour. They made money! They helped people lose weight! They helped the weak become stronger, and the youths become more athletic. They wore the distinct "Trainer" label on their shirts and they carried their own business cards! Soon, word of mouth was the best sales tactic they could use...client were referring friends and family! Results were being noted everywhere—in the gym, at family reunions, at church gatherings, in public, and in homes!

But then "*they* "came...
Yes, then the ones that had little or no experience came in. The ones that wanted all the glamour without working for it. The ones that thought their time was too valuable and demanded to be paid more. The ones that followed all the false prophet magazines. The ones that felt they were destined to be trainers.

I wrote this article because in 6 years of direct personal training and 3 years of direct management of personal trainers, I have had the opportunity to interview 43 *"wanna-be"* trainers in my career. Some were destined to be good trainers and I hired them, some were destined to waste my time. I have the opportunity to instruct classes on personal trainers in community colleges in Connecticut and each year, I meet over 100 new people wanting to become a personal trainer. I workout in 4 different clubs 3 times a week and I have the opportunity to observe trainers in action. I teach workshops on advanced strength training techniques for trainers 4 times a year and have the opportunity to speak to trainers in their first year *"on the job"*. I talk and I listen, and I realize that 50% of the trainers fail. Here are my top 5 reason why:

Trainers Think Their Time is <u>TOOO</u> valuable.

This one perturbs me to no end. Since when is your time to valuable to help someone? Many trainers charge up to $100 an hour for their time! I'm sorry but I would never pay anyone $100 for anything. Trainers tend to set their price based on what *"more important things they could be doing at the time of the session"* (playing with the kids, watching that DVD, making dinner, going out shopping, etc), rather than setting their price based on their level of expertise and background. Too many trainers want the Ferrari as soon as they get the driver's license. <u>Personal training is not a self-serving career.</u> You help others...you give yourself to others, you sacrifice crappy hours, and dealing with different personality types to help others. The time of the less fortunate (or less healthy in this case) is more valuable than ours...*because they don't have as much left as we do.*

Everyone Wants to Be a Trainer

This one I can feel for. Some people develop a desire to help others. I truly understand that testament to help another human in an unfavorable condition. But...just like everyone is not meant to be a doctor, lawyer, and astronaut—*neither is everyone meant to be a personal trainer just because you went through the Express line at your local gym for 12 weeks and lost 14 pounds.* That doesn't make you a professional. There is nothing wrong with wanting to be something in life...but to be good at what you do in this field is what separates you from everyone else.

Marketing Guru's Grant Everyone Permission to Call Themselves Trainers

Okay...over the last 2 years there has been an incredible influx of personal training studios, boot camps, websites, and products. This saturation has caused harm in the personal training industry. Many of these personal trainers are encouraged to market themselves and develop half-assed programs. Are they purposely developing half-assed programs? No...But that is the level of competence out there because they are focused more on making a buck through marketing and easy cash. So THEY are making tons of money off of these newbies. And potential clients don't know the difference. And another detrimental effect of all of this is: newbies are great at advertising, developing websites, and using sales strategies; but when it comes to training a client....they suck! So the client is "turned off" by the lack of experience, knowledge, professionalism, creativity, and responsibility by these newbies and guess what?

The field has been overly clogged with people wanting to share their services BEFORE they are actually good at them! "Our field is labeled a JOKE!

Trainers Don't Workout Themselves

I see this one from time to time. Trainers encouraging their clients to perform a one-arm, one leg standing cable row with rotation on a ½ foam roller! Well....I'm not going to get in to the fact that they trainer may not know exactly why he or she is performing that exercise. But I will get into the fact that I know for a fact—just by looking at the trainer—that the trainer does not perform or cannot perform that exercise. Why do trainers do this? Is it because such an exercise is hard and we want our client to suffer, or is it because the exercise has a purpose? So many trainers are out of shape and not conditioned for the type of training they prescribe (power-lifting, HIIT, functional, etc, etc...) Well, guess what? It's not only about being physically capable of performing the exercise, but it is more importantly about knowing "<u>where and how</u>" to cue the exercise and understand the mental skills required to perform the exercise. That is why if you preach it, you should practice it!

Trainers Don't Continue to Learn

I can't say this enough. To be in the position of developing exercise programs for sedentary people that put their hard-earned money and trust into you is so important. A doctor doesn't graduate school and start seeing patients---they perform a residency at a hospital...for years! Trainers must understand that this practice is more than holding a clipboard and counting reps...it is about understanding the human body and how it correlate to stresses your clients puts on it, and what physical stresses YOU put on it through exercise. An exercise program without modifications in its first 2 weeks is a joke to me. Any trainer that carries around the latest edition of Men's Fitness during a session is a joke to me. Any trainer that cannot admit that they need assistance or need to refer out is a joke to me. I have met trainers that were certified in 1988 and have not learned anything new. Do you know how much fitness has evolved in just 3 years? Half of today's trainers do not put the time, effort, and money into continuing education, seminars, or instructional books and videos. They want to make money and not invest in their skills or experience. Imagine this: If I sold you a computer with 2.5 Intel Pentium Processor® for $1200, wouldn't you be upset if you turned around and saw the same price tag on a computer with 4.0 Intel Pentium Processor®? You would want the faster computer because you were getting more for your money! Well, sorry to say, not every client is getting the most for their dollars. Some are paying trainers based on their looks, sales tactics, or not knowing what they are getting themselves into.

I don't mean for this article to offend anyone. I look at this article as a challenge for you to step it up. Personal training can be a dog-eat-dog career choice and if your intentions are placed correctly, you can enjoy a long successful career in it. Don't let this article discourage you, but let it awaken the original reasons why you want to be a trainer.

5 Small, But Crucial Cardio Mistakes
By John Izzo

Not Drinking Water During the Workout

My girlfriend is guilty of this. I notice that when we do our cardio training together, she never sips her water. The bottle just lays in its little cubby-hole on the cardio console and she gulps it down *at the end*. Did you hear what I said? *I said she GULPS it down at the end of the cardio session*. Hydration is so important, especially during strenuous physical activity, that even a 2% loss in hydration will affect performance. Dehydration, combined with strenuous exercise, creates an environment of not only physical, but mental stress. How does mental stress affect your performance? If you "feel" that you are over-exerting yourself, chances are you will not increase the level on your treadmill, cross trainer, bike, or stepper. Chances are as performance decreases, so will your drive to increase the power outage that you may be capable of doing. Hence, steady state cardio work prevails...

The lesson here? Take sips throughout your cardio session every other minute. There are various physical signs that you are beginning to experience dehydration during exercise: 1.) you cannot keep posture and composure during cardio exercise, 2.) your cheeks and face become rosey red and flushed, 3.) you do not sweat normally.

Doing the Same Cardio Machine Day After Day

I know why we all do this. We get good at what we started out doing! Just think 6 weeks ago, you thought level 5 on the elliptical trainer was impossible. Now you are continuously jumping up to level 7 with no difficulty whatsoever. That is a great accomplishment for the standard sedentary individual who has finally adapted daily exercise into their lives and has made some improvements in body composition and overall health. BUT...for the typical hard gainer, this is a carnival merry-go-round. Typically, we need to feel successful to justify the work we put into improving our bodies, increasing strength, or losing fat. I have always said that "success breeds success". So psychologically, when we "get good" on a particular type of cardiovascular activity (i.e. running, elliptical, rowing, stepper, etc), we tend to believe that we have reached a pinnacle in our training. That's not a bad thing. But again, for the hard gainer, this can be a vicious cycle of nothingness. This cycle is a result of the body's specific adaptation to imposed demands (SAID) principle. The hardest exercise becomes easier the better we get at it. Therefore, the better we are at it, the more efficient we become at that particular activity. The more efficient we become at the activity, the less calories we burn. (*Read that again if you do not understand*) Oh yea...forget the little calorie counter that pops up on the screen. It's based on total weight and keeps going even when you step on the sides of the treadmill.

Steady State Cardio

We all heard how this one is a waste of time. Let me explain how it is a waste of time in regards to fat loss. The body uses 3 sources of energy to sustain ATP (adenosine tri-phosphate) production. ATP is the body's end-all, be-all source of energy. In order for the body to live, it must continuously produce ATP. Well, it does this in 3 ways. Our immediate source of energy production comes from creatine phosphate (CP), where a creatine molecule is donated to ADP (adenosine di-phosphate) to create ATP. This action is **anaerobic** and requires only creatine which the body supplies or is obtained from meats. This immediate source of energy lasts only around 5 seconds and is primarily used for power. The second source of energy is glycolosis—the breaking down of sugars to produce ATP. This process is also **anaerobic** and lasts usually 3 to 5 minutes. Glycolysis refers to the body using glycogen (stored sugar) in blood and muscles to continuously make ATP. This process is the one we usually exercise in. The third and often never tapped into is oxidative phosphorilization. This process is **aerobic** and calls upon oxygen to aid in mobilizing fat cells to be used as energy. This process allows the body to last longer in endurance type bouts or high intense bouts of exercise. So...how does this correlate with steady state exercise? Easy. When we perform 30 minutes of walking, we never step out of glycolosis as our primary source of ATP production (energy). We are simply burning off the sugars of foods we have eaten in the last 24-48 hours. We never try to sprint on the treadmill, pick the higher level on the elliptical, or take a spinning class...we basically do what we have been taught or what comes easiest. This has been my argument in regards to watching TV while doing cardio. If your goal is fat loss, you can try the steady state stuff for a while, but when your cardiovascular system improves and your diet is better, then you need to work harder to expedite oxidative phosphorilization. This fat mobilizing process is also known as EPOC (Excessive Post- Exercise Oxygen Consumption). In simple terms it means that the body continues to mobilize fat as fuel for up to 1 hour **after** an intense bout of cardio (180+ bpm).

Afraid to Do Cardio Before Weights

This is an old bodybuilder's myth that started way back when. Why do we think cardio (the right kind—not steady state) will cause muscle loss? It is okay to perform your cardio BEFORE your strength training—even if your goal is hypertrophy or strength. Why? Because if you follow the proper food intake and understand the amount of calories you need to sustain lean body mass, than intense bouts of cardio (defined as above 180+ bpm, short duration (12-15minutes)) will actually promote muscle gain. The real fear should come from figuring out the total amount of calories you ingested for a 24 hour period. This is what I used to tell my clients...ever see a sprinter? Ever see how muscular they are?

Doing your cardio first and then performing strength training can lead to the EPOC phenomenon that I mentioned above. Of course, this is dependent on your intensity, rep schemes, rest periods, and fitness level.

Old Sneakers

There is no doubt in my mind that 70% of foot and knee problems come from poor or old sneakers. How many times have you seen gym-goers running on the treadmill with old, beat-up sneakers with grass stains, and cracks all over the "p-leather"? I mean, those sneakers are used for Saturday morning lawn mowing and then taken to the gym to perform your 30 minutes cardio routine? C'mon....

In the last 4 years, every client that I met that had old sneakers evidenced by the condition, wear of soles, and or "lack of bounce", I had them purchase new ones. I would not start their training program until they came to me with new sneakers. Period. You know what happened? Knee pain disappeared...foot pain disappeared...and clients didn't cut cardio out of their workouts. They felt better running or doing inclines. You know that pain you feel on the elliptical in your foot? It disappeared with a brand new pair of Adidas®. How does sneaker condition affect lower body function? If your soles are worn, or your have pronated or supinated ankles, chances are your foot strike is not optimal on hard surfaces or a treadmill. What this does is create dysfunction at the ankle joint (usually due to dynamic instability) and weak/tight peroneals and tibialis (ankle muscles). This kinetic chain dysfunction travels up to the next joint, which is the knee and then the hip and causes undue stress on the lower back and entire spinal column. This is another reason why people skip out on cardio or like the steady state easy stuff—because their feet can't handle it! Besides, a new pair of sneakers gives people the sense of starting something new and committing to a fitness program.

5 Annoying Problems in Gyms Across the US
By John Izzo

1.) *"Functional Equipment Being Used for Bodybuilding Exercises"*

I guess this is more or less a pet peeve, or it can be viewed as a lack of variation in exercise selection. How many times have you walked around your fitness center and marveled at all the new functional equipment that it had? **I classify functional equipment as any cable apparatus that has moveable arms, pulleys, or is multi-vector** *(most notably Free Motion®, Paramount®, Keiser®, and some Precor®, Life Fitness® and other reputable equipment manufacturers).* So, the most annoying thing to see in the gym with this arsenal of movement improving equipment is some guy performing your typical cable crossovers or double biceps curls. We have all seen him (or her). The selection of functional exercises that can be performed due to the mobility and angles at which each pulley can be placed is numerous. But why perform your typical sagital plane crossovers? Are the cable towers occupied? Is your chest workout incomplete without the crossover exercise? Is this the idea of variation from say...the peck deck machine? Obviously, there is lack of knowledge of the usage of these pieces. Although, crossovers and double-bi curls can be performed on them, why choose to do it on a machine that is designed for multi-planar functionality? Learn more exercises!

2.) "Too-Wide-of-a-Grip Lat Pull-Downs"

Unless you are 6'2" and above, there is no reason to go wide on your lat pull down grip. The old fallacy of "go wider—get a wider back; or "go narrow—get a thicker back" are exactly that: **old bodybuilding fallacy.** According to the NASM, using a wider grip actually brings in more scapular movement and involvement (which it is involved during the movement) but the majority of work comes from abduction of the scapula and rhomboids---not the lats. The lats are what you want to work together with strong scapular retraction and depression. Also, going too wide of a grip also tends the lifter to constantly elevate the shoulder blades with each rep. The proper way to perform the lat pull down is with shoulder blades depressed down and kept in that position throughout the set. We tend to raise our shoulder blades and thoracic spine because these muscles are eccentrically weak. Thus, we should focus on strengthening the scapular retractors/protractors and stabilizers to perform a perfect lat pull down.

3.) "Medicine Balls Used for Crunches"

I don't know if this one is me...Vern Gambetta popularized a lot of medicine ball movements in the mid-1990's including wood-chops, oblique twists, and lunge twists. Medicine balls have become so popular that they are also manufactured with handles! In my opinion, and hopefully other strength coaches, weighted medicine balls should be used primarily for power movements **--aka: throwing against a concrete wall to maximize power output of a specific movement: chest pass (soccer throw); oblique transverse passes (tennis racquet), vertical leaps (basketball dunk), and many more).**

I have a problem with this vital tool being used by many gym-goers across the US as a way to load the ab crunch. We have all seen them....guy or girl gets on the bench or ball and holds the med ball overhead with straight arms and crunches. *Is a dumbbell not sufficed for this movement?* Did you know we used to use dumbbells for stuff like this before med balls were ever in gyms? The only thing is we couldn't throw dumbbells or we got thrown out of the gym! Medicine balls are designed to be thrown—to take a beating—witnessed by the material they are made up! Use them for what they should primarily be used for: Power!

4.)   *"Boyfriends Teaching Their Girlfriends How To Lift"*

I am guilty of this, but I hopefully know what I am talking about. Every week, I spot half a dozen couples working out together and they are made up of big buff guys teaching their *"pilates-addicted"* girlfriends ***"how they work out"***. So what is wrong with this? Many guys who are in between the ages of 25-45 have grown up with watching the likes of Arnold, Dorian, Lee, and Ronnie (pro-bodybuilders). So if you are like me, you grew up wanting to be big, strong, and cut. Well, if you subscribed to all the magazines like I did, you learned a lot of the sagital plane exercises from the bodybuilding sample routines. So flash-forward to the present day: boyfriends teach their girlfriends the bench press, lat pull-down, bent-over row, lateral raises, squat, leg press, curls, kickbacks, and many more. **So girlfriends begin training like men who train like bodybuilders.** What is wrong with that? Nothing...but if you know conventional bodybuilding routines you'll know that they contain a lot of sagital presses and most bodybuilders have the resulted syndromes of such training: upper and lower-cross syndrome & protracted shoulders. So why are you going to mess up your girlfriend's body? The solution ladies? Seek out a qualified fitness professional to show you how to perform an abundance of multi-planar exercises including bodyweight, bands, balls, and core work. Don't pass up the free session that you get upon joining a gym. It is your opportunity to ask questions and be instructed on the proper way to perform a **variety of exercises**. Back in the day, when a woman said *"I don't want to look like one of those bodybuilding people"*, **now I know what they meant.**

5.) *"TVs in front of Cardio Equipment"*

I can write an entire article on this and I probably will. Managing a YMCA fitness center for the last 2 years, I have found the reason why people are not losing fat. They are coming **into the gym to watch TV and workout.** *Did you hear what I said?* They <u>are coming in to watch TV and workout</u>. You and I go to the gym to work out and maybe, if "Rescue Me™" is on... watch TV. Today's general population clientele (GPC) has misunderstood what exercise is thanks to the ACSM. People pick the cross trainer or treadmill in front of a TV, plug in their headphones, put on their favorite show and walk at a 2.5 pace. After a half hour, they have not even broken a sweat and their cardio session is complete. They feel content because, according to present-day guidelines, they just achieved an important factor in their longevity and got to watch the latest episode of "24™". Their real intent is to pay attention to the show on TV and walk. To pay attention to the show, they need to walk at a reasonable pace that will not cause them focus on maintaining balance, endurance, and effort. **The very things needed to generate power output to expend the most calories in the least amount of time, thus losing fat!** I am not saying this is the majority of gym-goers, but it is what I witness 80% of the time. It is to no surprise that many of the people I witnessed still look the same year after year. Fitness centers need to get rid of all these TV's and cardio theater systems in front of cardio equipment and focus more on member goal attainment and not dollar signs.

Also Available by the Author:

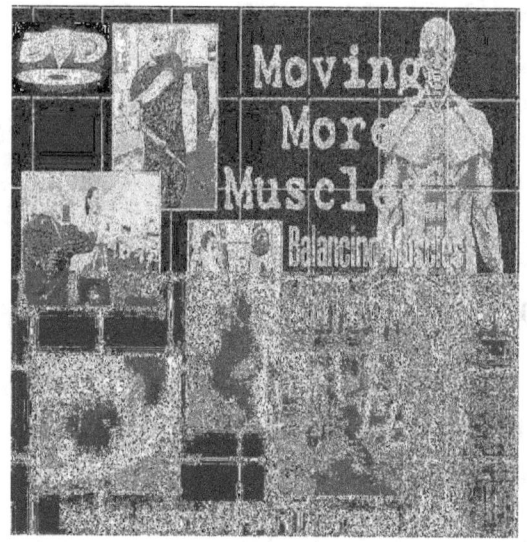

Moving More Muscles DVD

Learn how to balance muscle groups by creating efficient exercise programs utilizing push & pull combination sets. The video is over one hour long and contains dozens of new exercises including core, mobility, and power movements. A great video for those looking to take their workouts to another level. Available at www.standAPARTfitness.com.

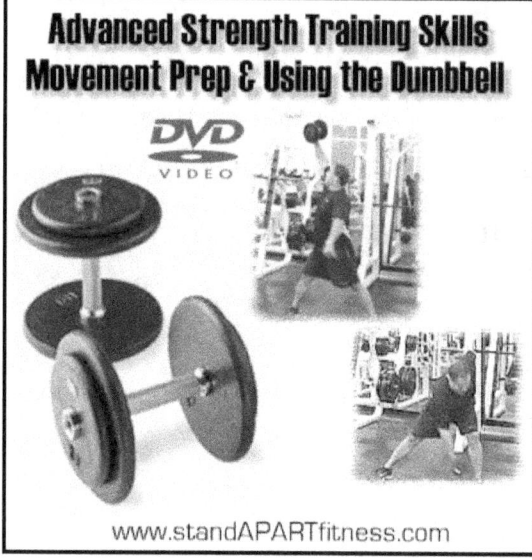

Advanced Strength Training Techniques DVD: *Movement Prep & Using the Dumbbell*

This DVD features numerous exercises that utilize the core, upper body and lower body —with just dumbbells! Includes a mobility drill warm-up and is jam packed with advanced moves. Perfect for anyone who works out in their homes or travels. Available at www.standAPARTfitness.com.

More DVDs available at:

www.standAPARTfitness.com

Daily exercise tips and daily personal trainer tasks discussed at:

http://lifeofapersonaltrainer.blogspot.com

www.ingramcontent.com/pod-product-compliance
Lightning Source LLC
Chambersburg PA
CBHW052005280526
45793CB00005B/858